Diabetes United

By Raymah Bryant, 11-Year-Old CEO

Contents

Foreword

Welcome to "Diabetes United," a cookbook dedicated to all the young and aspiring chefs who, like me, manage diabetes while living life to the fullest. My name is Raymah Bryant, and I'm excited to share my journey and recipes with you. Living with diabetes doesn't mean you have to miss out on delicious and nutritious meals. Together, we'll explore tasty dishes that help maintain our health and happiness.

Introduction

I'm Raymah Bryant, an 11-year-old who loves volleyball, dancing, and cooking healthy meals. Managing my diabetes with mindfulness and practicing good habits has helped me become a successful leader at home and school. This book is a collection of my favorite recipes that use quality ingredients and are designed to be diabetes-friendly.

I'm going into 6th grade and spend my summers going to Volleyball camp at Rogers Athletic Center (RAC) in Rogers, Arkansas, and Camp Aldersgate in Little Rock, Arkansas, with my friends. I moved from Shiloh Christian School in Springdale, Arkansas, after 3rd grade to find a more inclusive environment for my diabetes care and academics. My mother is my biggest cheerleader and mentor, and my stepmother, who is gluten-free, has taught me a lot about dietary restrictions. My dad and I enjoy practicing yoga, and I go fishing with my stepdad. All these activities keep me balanced and healthy.

Start your day with a nutritious and energizing breakfast! These recipes will give you the boost you need to tackle your morning activities with vigor.

Recipes:

Berry Good Morning Smoothie

- o Ingredients: **Fresh berries, Greek yogurt, chia seeds, almond milk, honey.**

- o Directions: **Blend all ingredients until smooth. Serve chilled.**

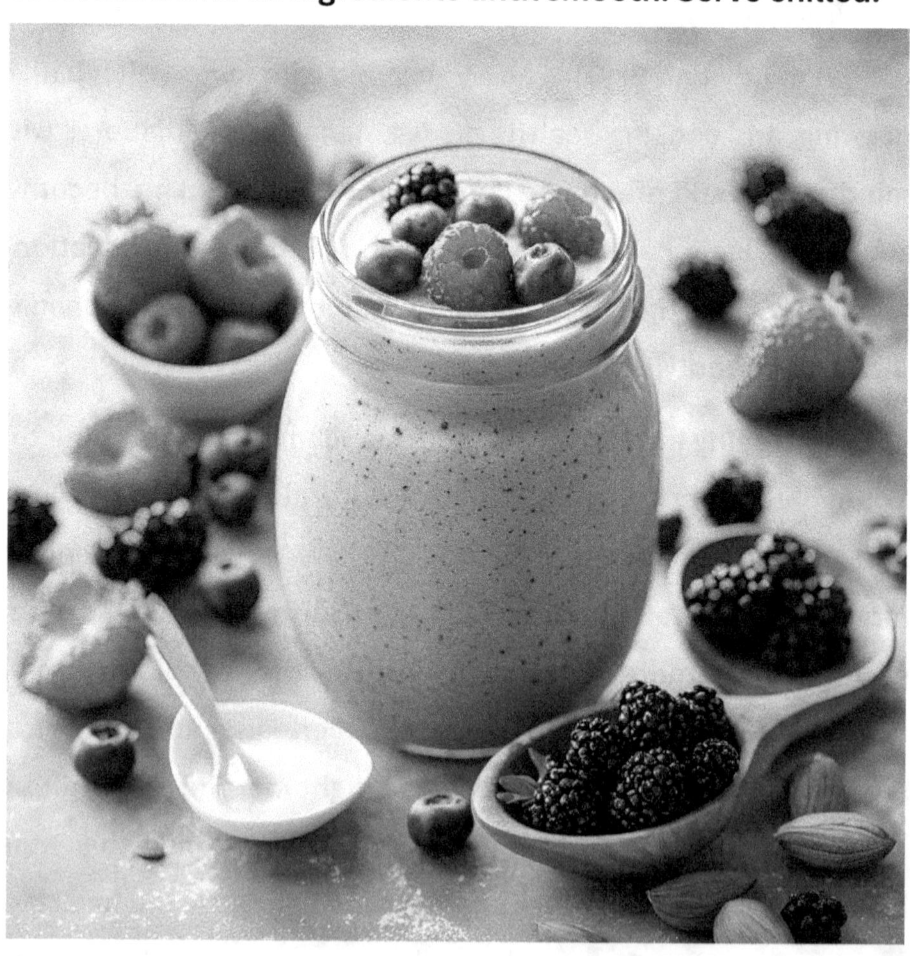

Veggie Omelette

- Ingredients: **Eggs, spinach, bell peppers, onions, tomatoes, cheese.**
- Directions: **Sauté veggies, whisk eggs, pour over veggies, cook until done, add cheese.**

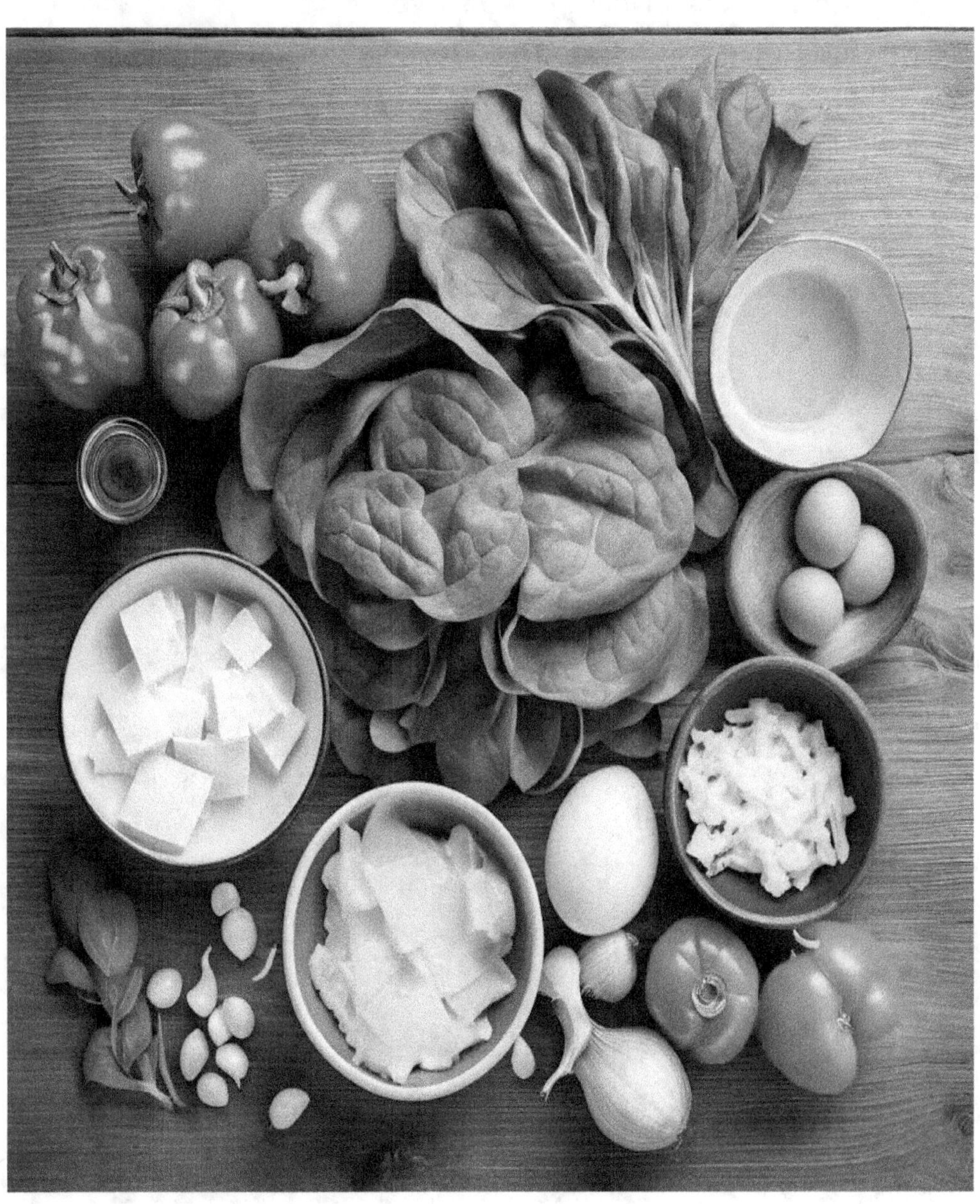

Gluten-Free Pancakes

- o Ingredients: **Gluten-free flour, almond milk, eggs, baking powder, vanilla extract.**

- o Directions: **Mix ingredients, pour batter on a hot griddle, cook until bubbles form, flip, and serve.**

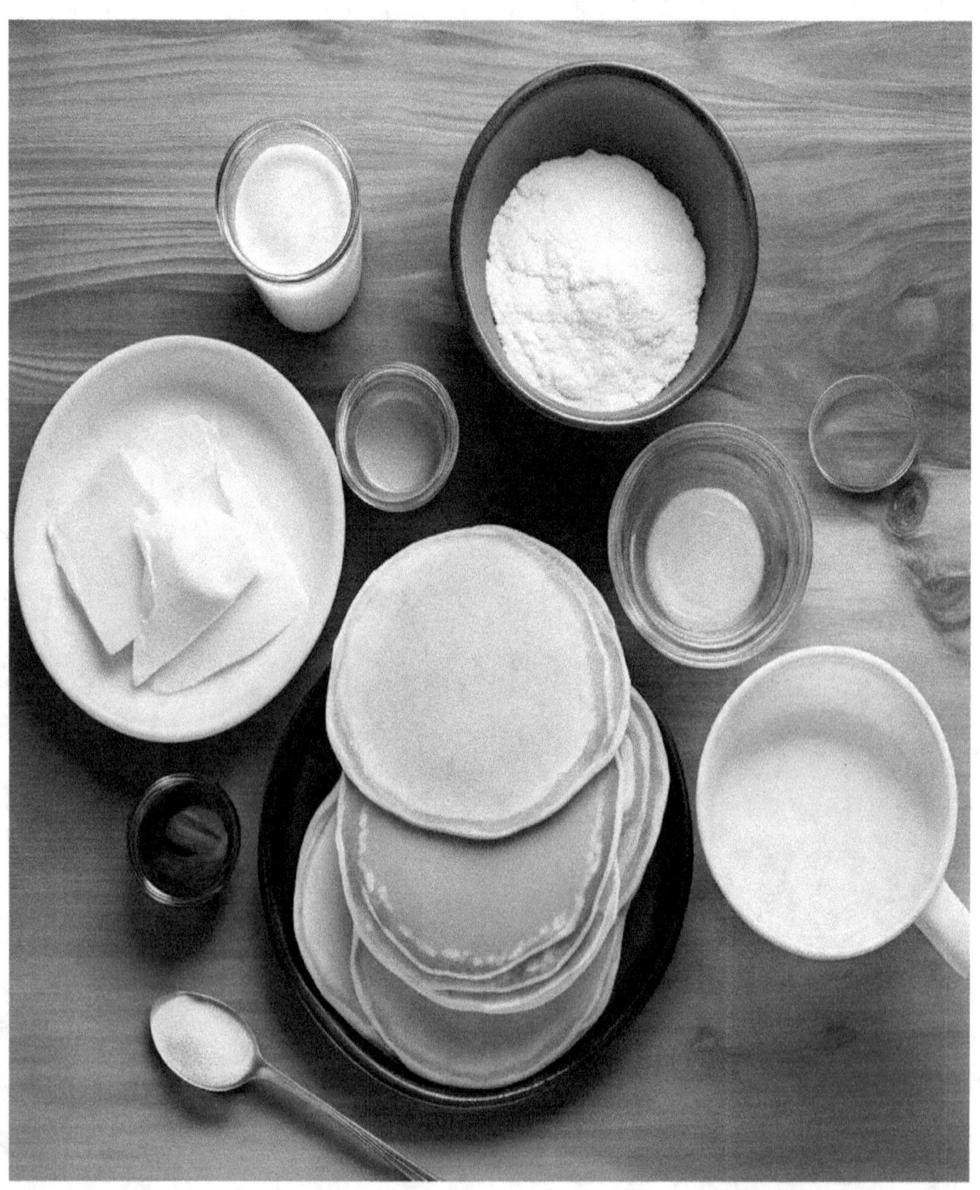

Morning Yoga Routine

- o **Start your day with a 15-minute yoga session with your family. Focus on stretches and poses that energize your body and mind.**

Nature Walk

- o **Take a brisk walk in your neighborhood or a nearby park. Enjoy the fresh air and observe the beauty of nature. This is a great way to clear your mind and prepare for the day ahead.**

Dance Party

- o **Put on your favorite music and dance around your living room. Dancing is a fun way to get your heart pumping and start your day on a positive note.**

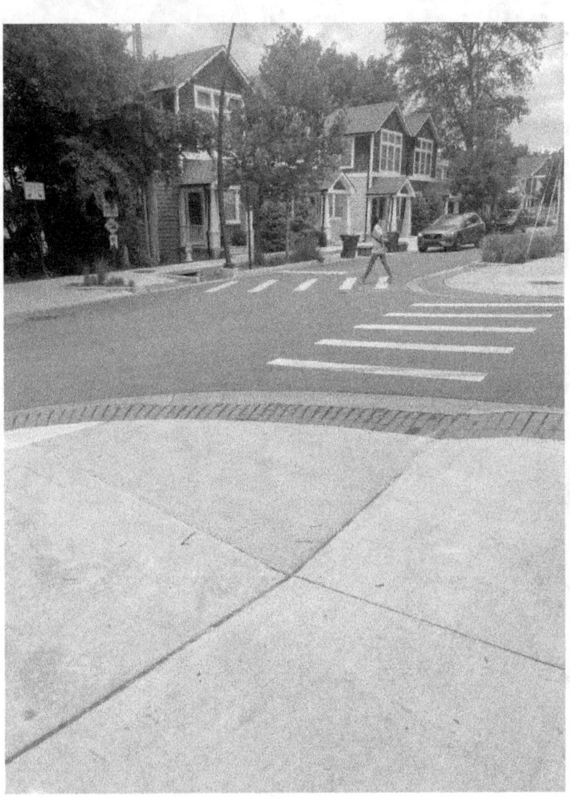

Keep your energy levels up throughout the day with these healthy and delicious snacks. Perfect for school breaks or after-school activities.

Recipes:

Hummus and Veggie Sticks

- o Ingredients: **Carrots, celery, bell peppers, hummus.**
- o Directions: **Slice veggies, serve with hummus for dipping.**

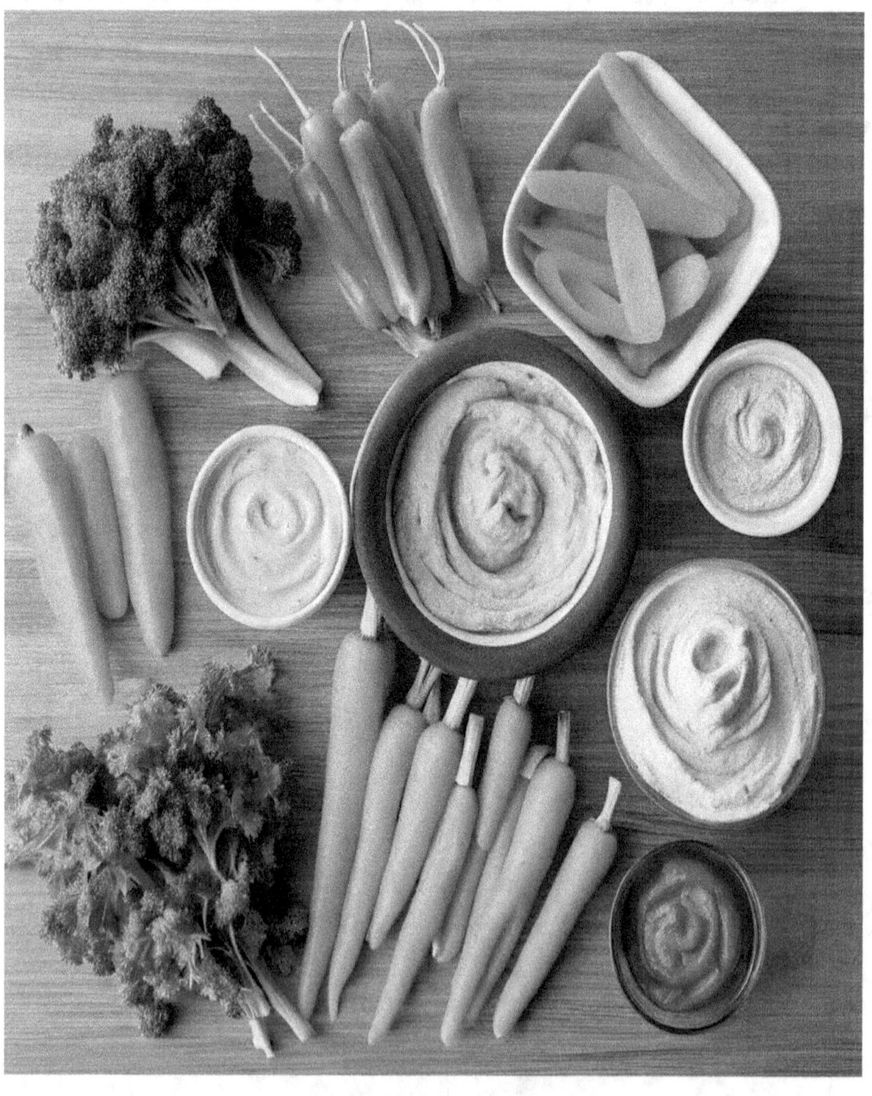

Fruit and Nut Mix

- o Ingredients: **Almonds, walnuts, dried cranberries, dark chocolate chips.**

- o Directions: **Mix all ingredients and store in an airtight container.**

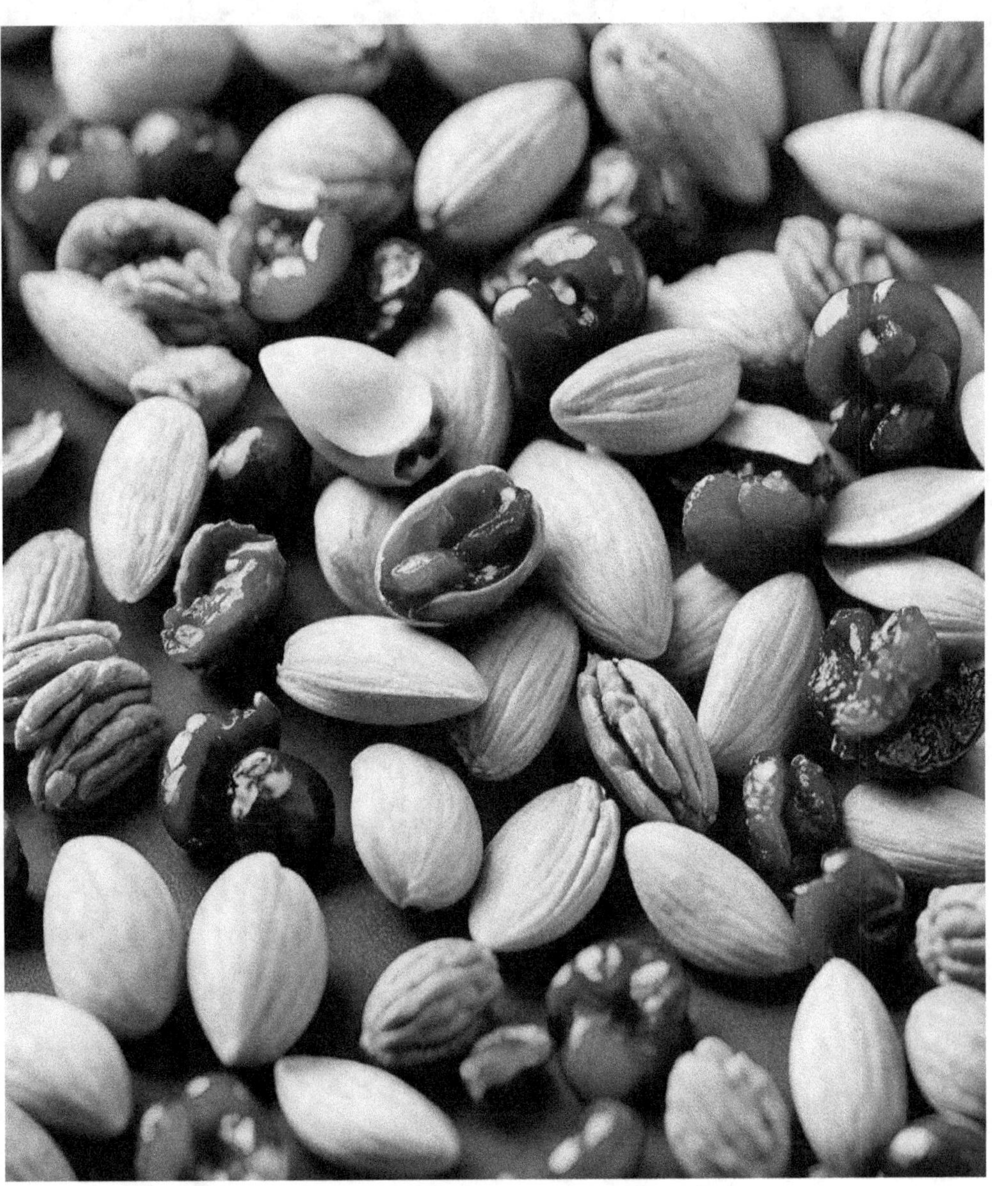

Apple Slices with Peanut Butter

- o Ingredients: **Apple slices, natural peanut butter.**

- o Directions: **Spread peanut butter on apple slices.**

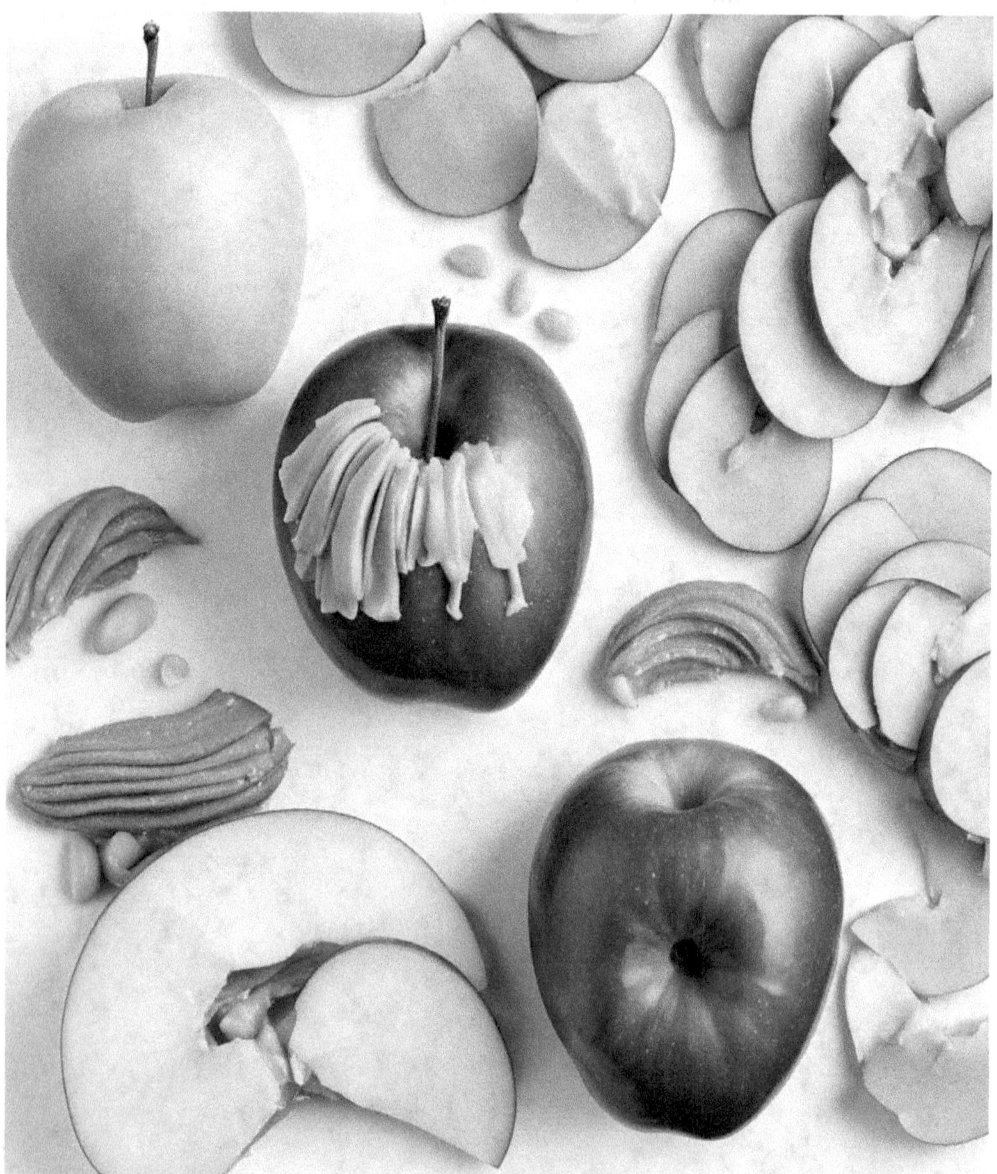

Brain Breaks

- o **Take short breaks during your study sessions to recharge. Do a quick puzzle, stretch, or take a few deep breaths to refresh your mind.**

Schoolyard Games

- o **Play games like tag, hopscotch, or jump rope with your friends during recess. These activities keep you active and help you stay focused in class.**

Creative Crafts

- o **Engage in a fun craft project, like making friendship bracelets or drawing. This is a great way to relax and express your creativity.**

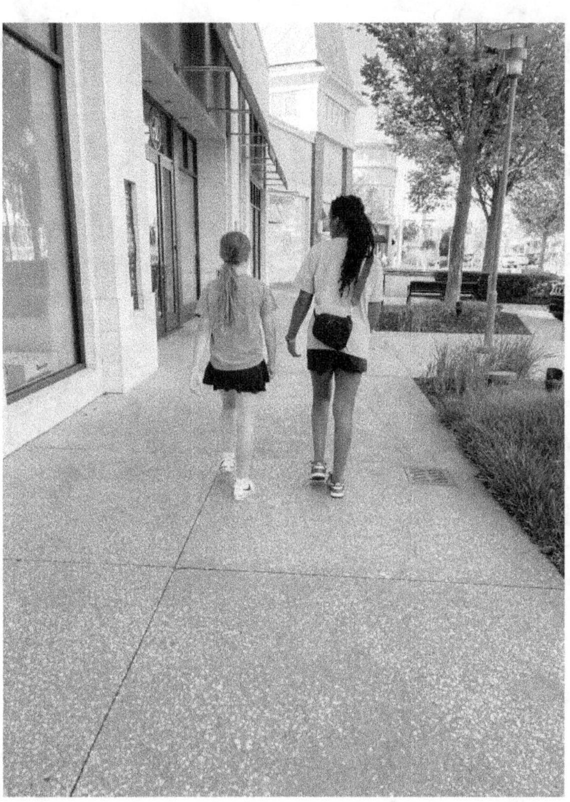

Fuel your afternoon with nutritious and satisfying lunches that keep you going strong. These recipes are perfect for school or at home.

Recipes:

Quinoa Salad

- o Ingredients: **Quinoa, cucumbers, cherry tomatoes, feta cheese, olive oil, lemon juice.**

- o Directions: **Cook quinoa, chop veggies, mix all ingredients together, and drizzle with olive oil and lemon juice.**

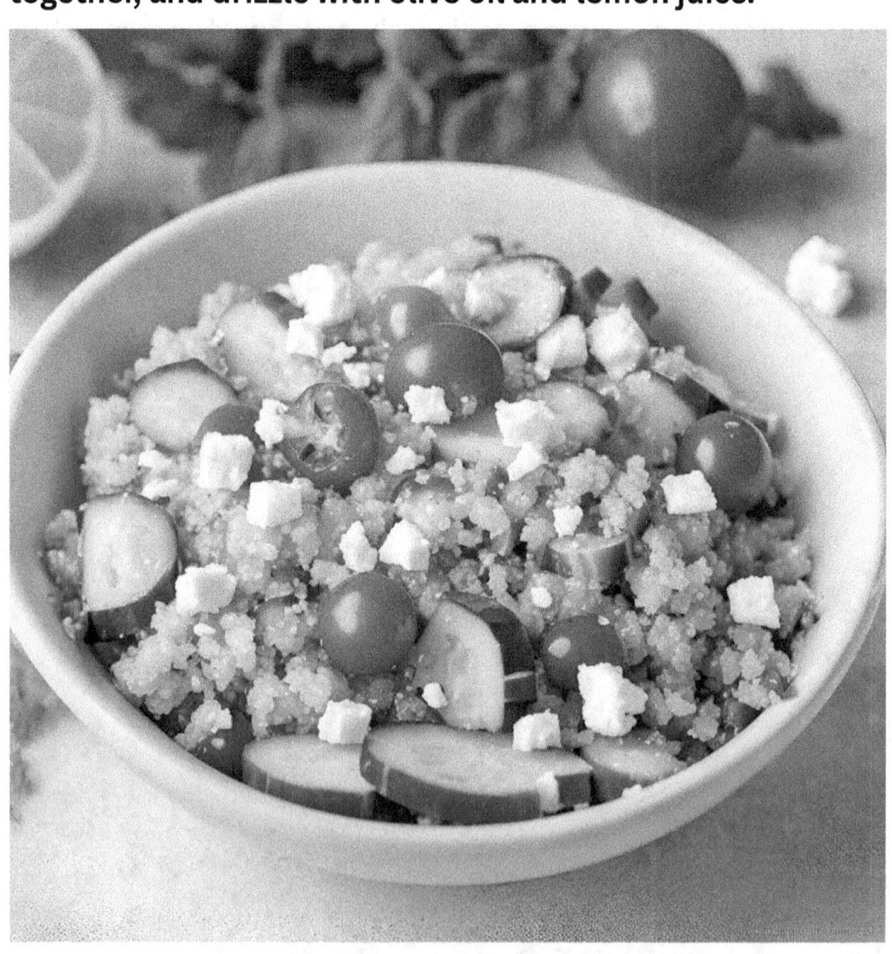

Turkey and Avocado Wrap

- o Ingredients: **Whole grain wrap, turkey slices, avocado, spinach, hummus.**
- o Directions: **Spread hummus on the wrap, add turkey, avocado, and spinach, then roll up.**

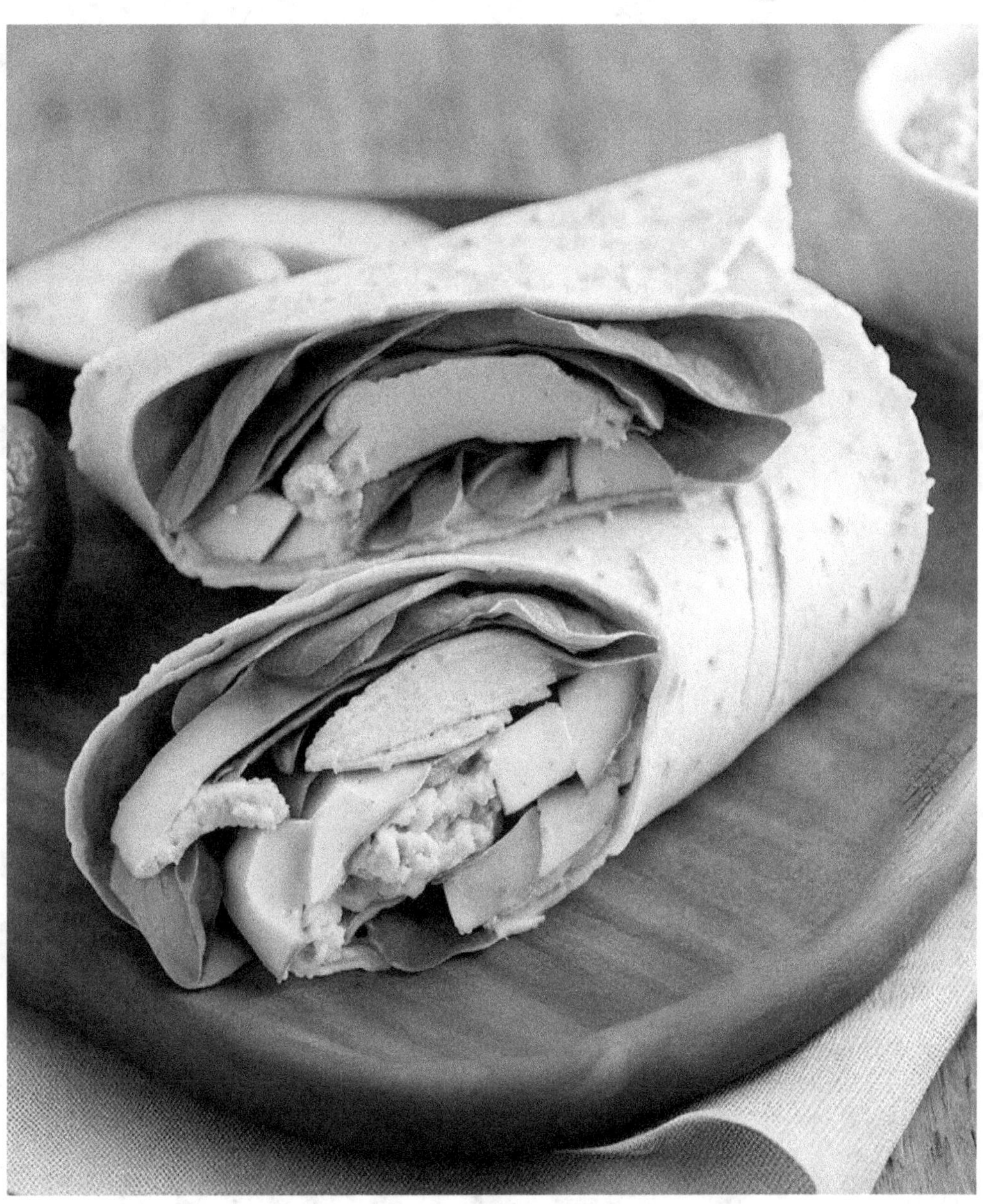

Gluten-Free Pasta Salad

- Ingredients: **Gluten-free pasta, olives, cherry tomatoes, mozzarella balls, basil, olive oil.**
- Directions: **Cook pasta, chop veggies, mix all ingredients, and toss with olive oil.**

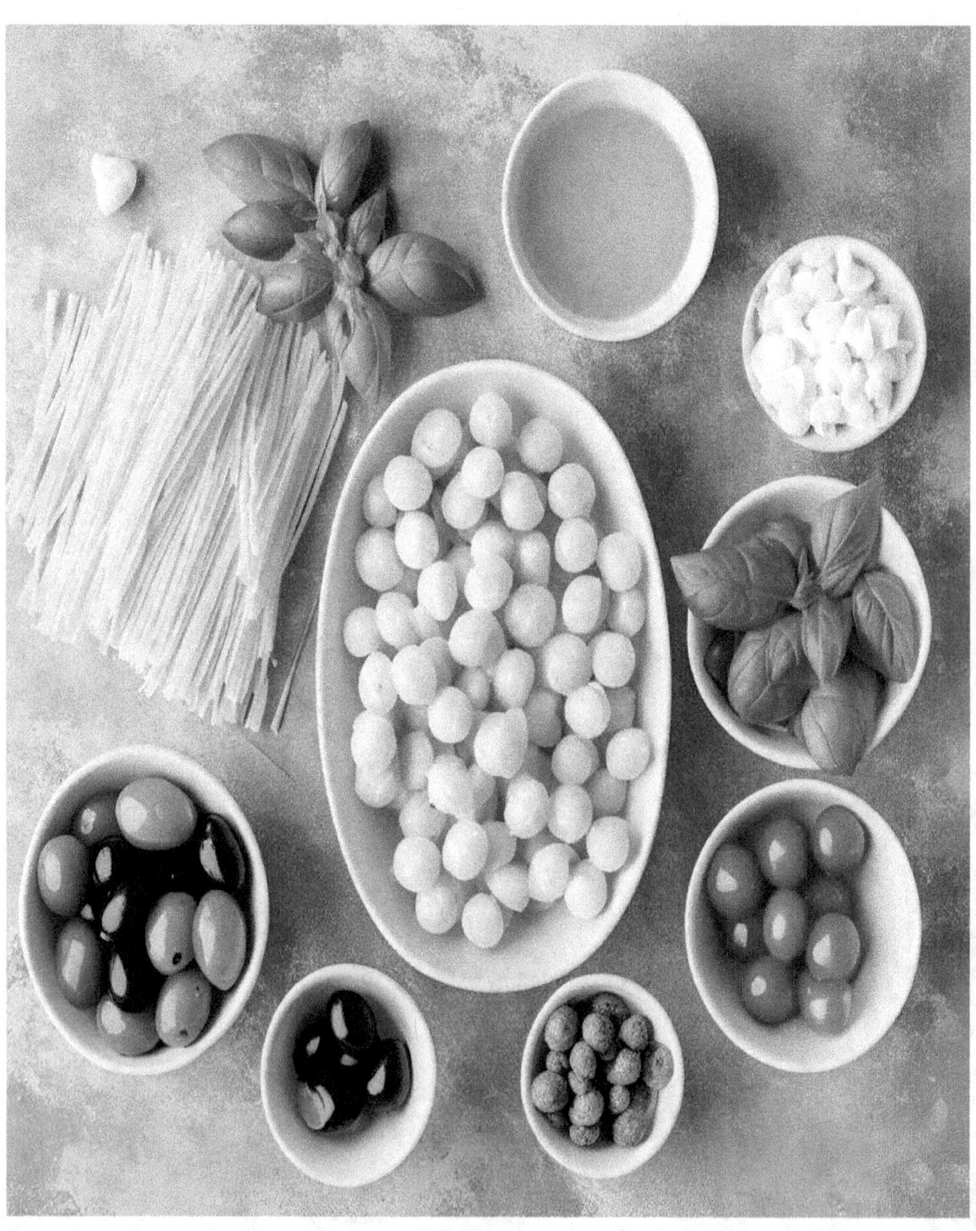

Activities:

Lunchtime Chats

- o **Have lunch with your friends or family and talk about your day. Sharing meals and conversations helps build strong relationships.**

Outdoor Play

- o **After lunch, spend some time playing outside. Activities like playing catch, riding your bike, or exploring nature are great ways to stay active.**

Mindful Eating

- o **Practice mindful eating by paying attention to your food's flavors, textures, and aromas. This helps you appreciate your meal and recognize when you're full.**

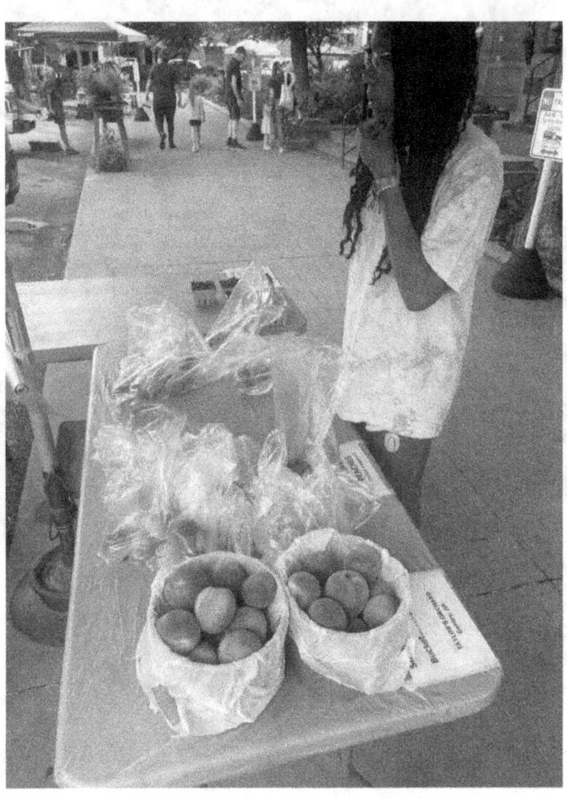

End your day with a hearty and healthy dinner that nourishes your body and mind. These recipes are perfect for family meals.

Recipes:

Grilled Chicken with Veggies

- Ingredients: **Chicken breasts, zucchini, bell peppers, olive oil, garlic, herbs.**
- Directions: **Marinate chicken with olive oil, garlic, and herbs, grill with veggies until cooked.**

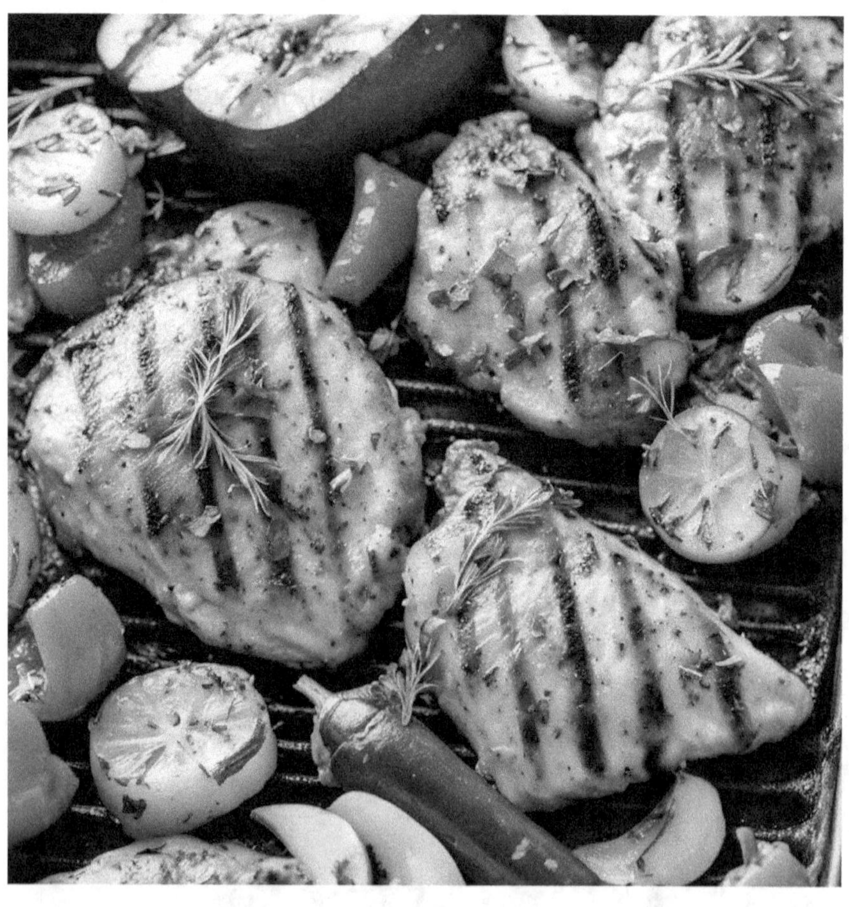

Baked Salmon

- o   Ingredients: **Salmon fillets, lemon, dill, olive oil, garlic.**
- o   Directions: **Preheat oven, place salmon on a baking sheet, drizzle with olive oil, lemon juice, garlic, and dill, bake until done.**

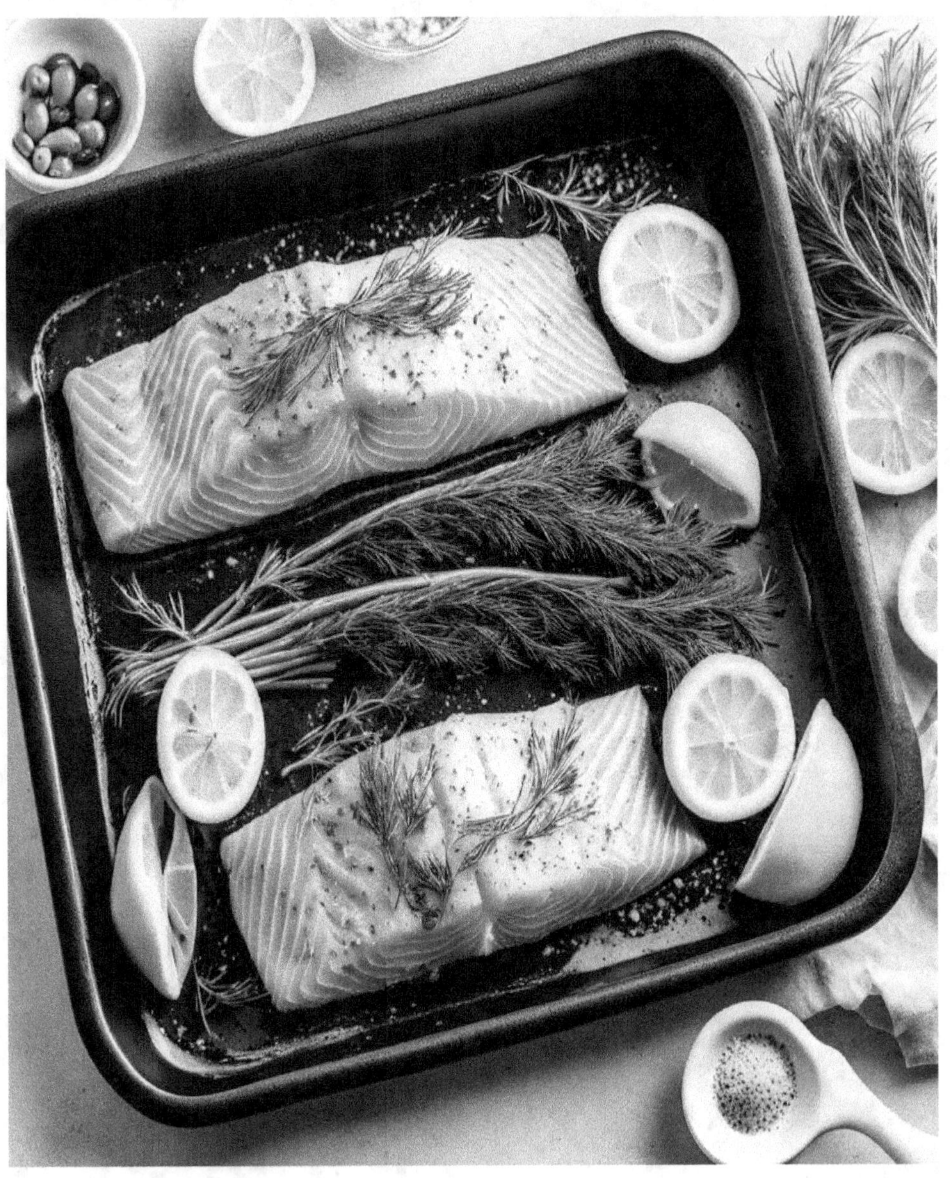

Stuffed Bell Peppers

- o Ingredients: **Bell peppers, ground turkey, quinoa, tomatoes, onions, cheese.**
- o Directions: **Cook turkey with onions, mix with quinoa and tomatoes, stuff into bell peppers, top with cheese, and bake.**

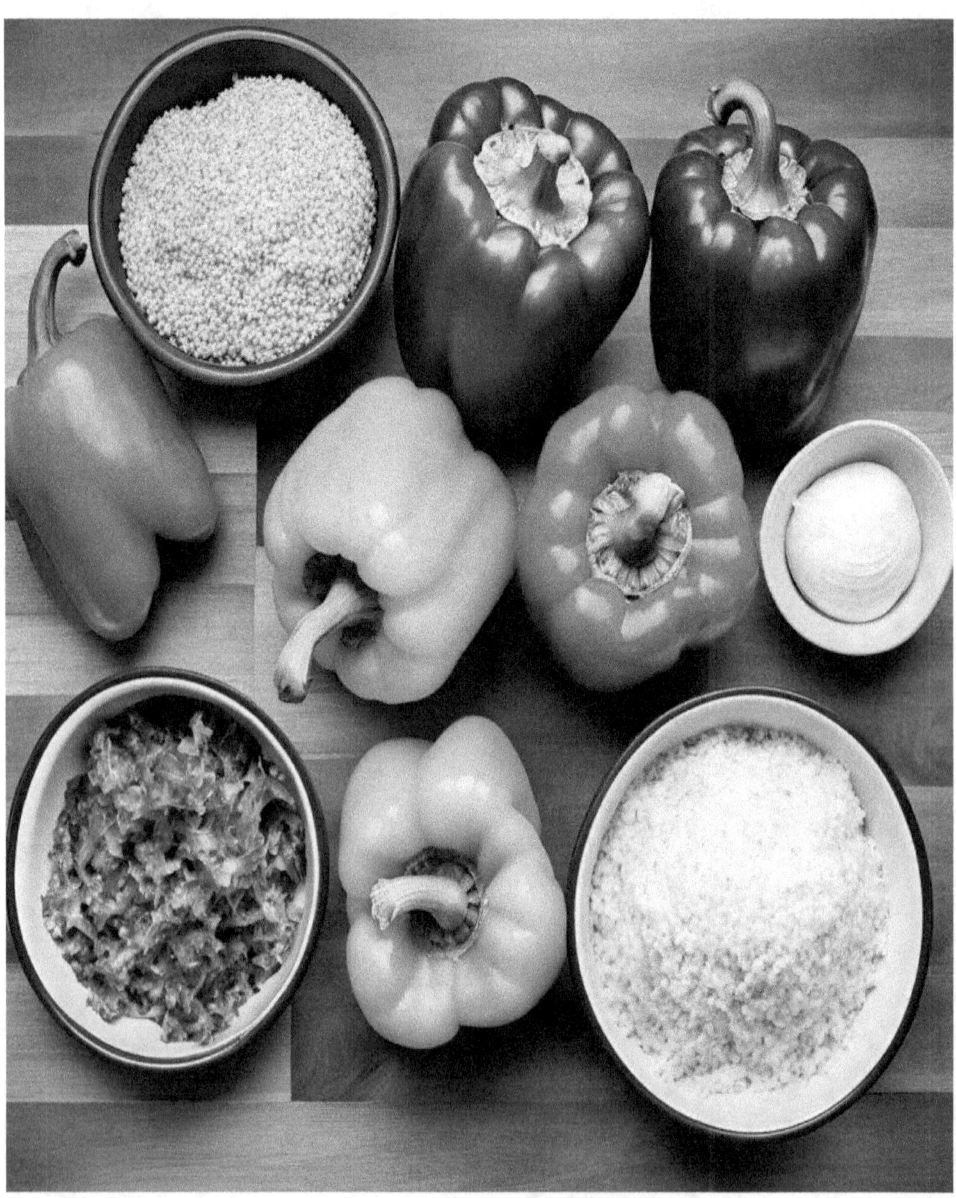

Activities:

Family Cooking Night

- **Cook dinner together as a family. Each member can help with different tasks, making it a fun and collaborative activity.**

Evening Walk

- **Take a walk after dinner to help with digestion and enjoy some quality time with your family.**

Reading Time

- **After dinner, spend some time reading your favorite book. This helps you relax and wind down for the night.**

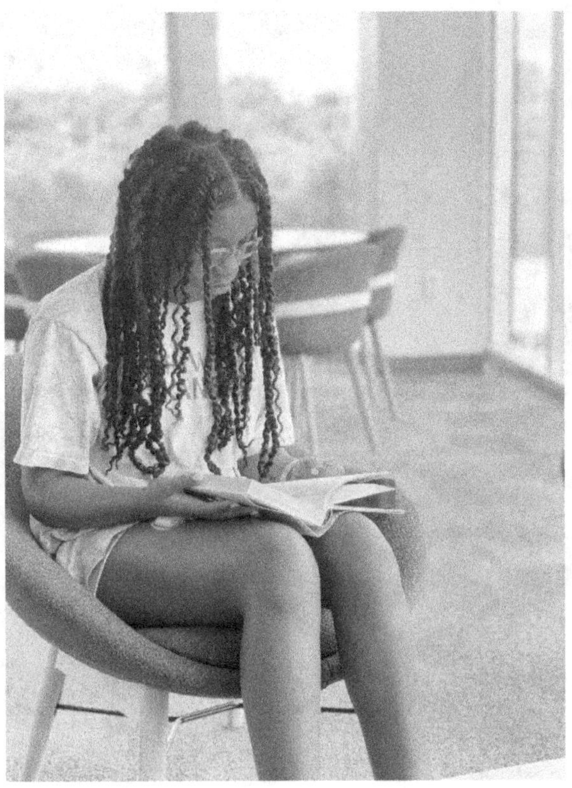

Indulge in these healthy and diabetes-friendly sweet treats that satisfy your cravings without compromising your health.

Recipes:

Greek Yogurt Parfait

- o Ingredients: **Greek yogurt, honey, granola, fresh berries.**
- o Directions: **Layer yogurt, honey, granola, and berries in a glass.**

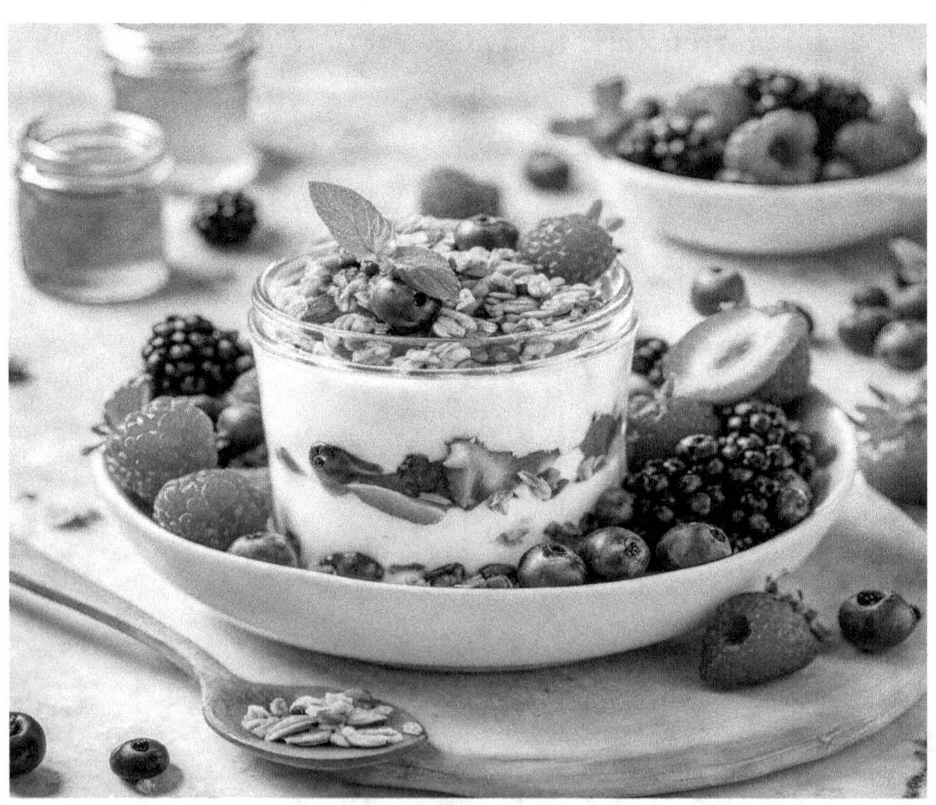

Dark Chocolate Avocado Mousse

- o Ingredients: **Avocados, dark chocolate, cocoa powder, honey, vanilla extract.**
- o Directions: **Blend all ingredients until smooth, chill before serving.**

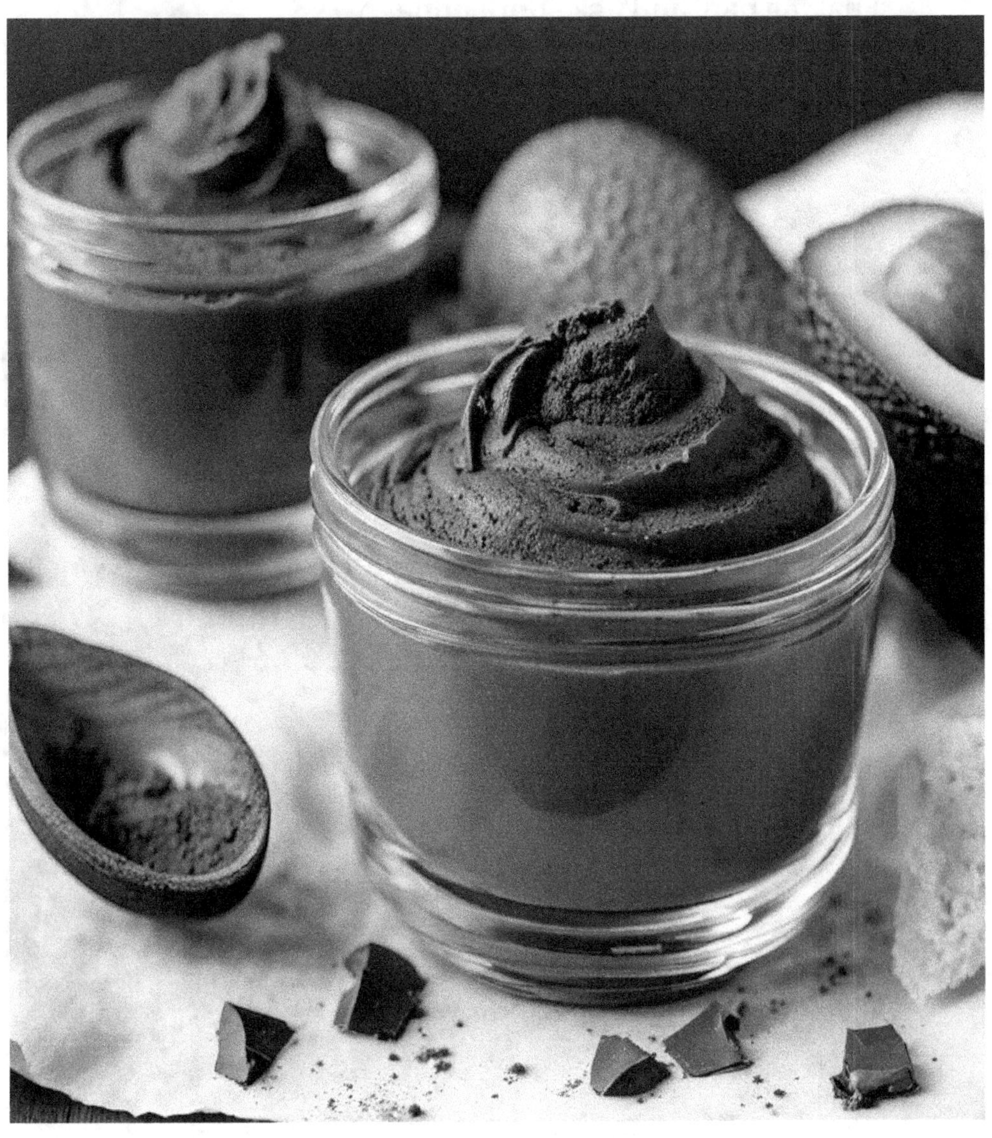

Gluten-Free Banana Bread

- o Ingredients: **Gluten-free flour, ripe bananas, eggs, baking soda, vanilla extract.**

- o Directions: **Mash bananas, mix with other ingredients, pour into a baking pan, and bake until done.**

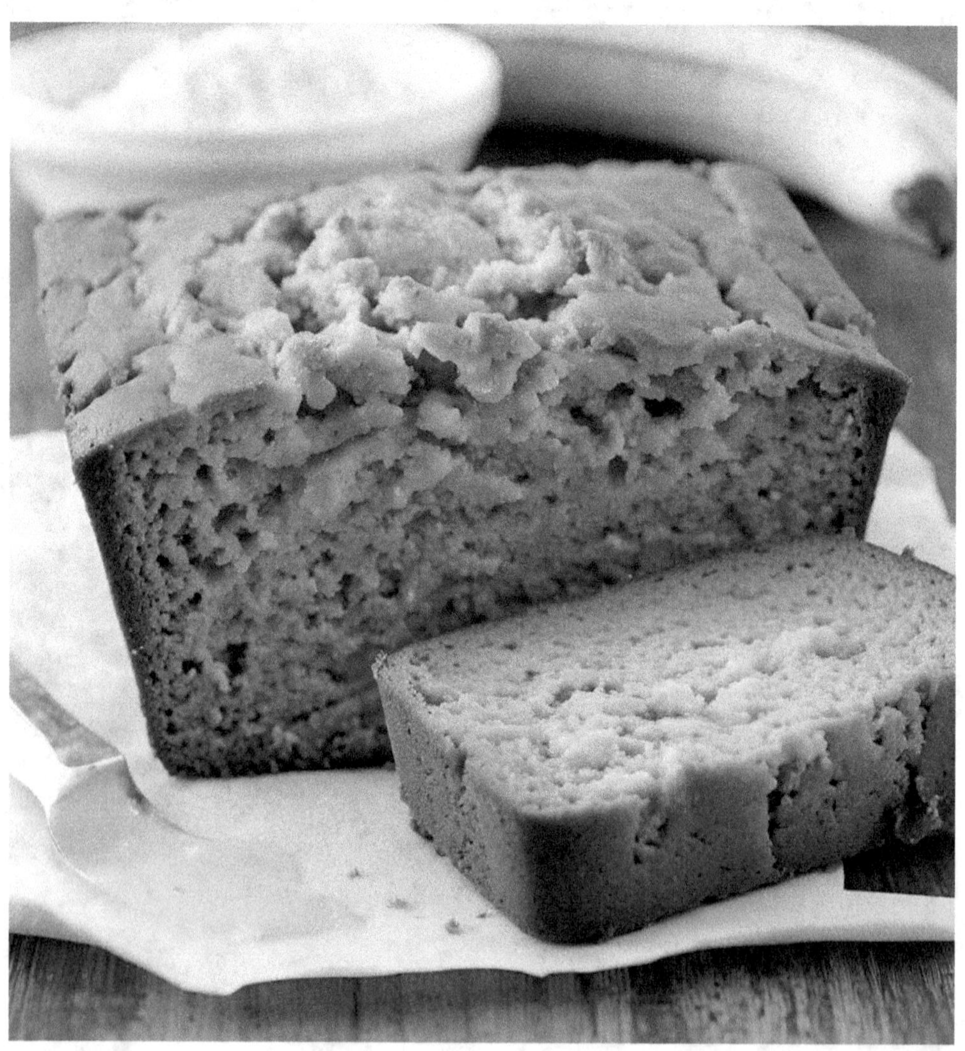

Activities:

Baking with Friends

- o **Invite your friends over for a baking session. It's a fun way to bond and share healthy treats.**

Mindful Desserts

- o **Enjoy your dessert slowly, savoring each bite. This practice of mindful eating helps you appreciate the flavors and eat in moderation.**

Gratitude Journaling

- o **After enjoying your sweet treat, take a few minutes to write in your gratitude journal. Reflecting on the positive aspects of your day helps foster a positive mindset.**

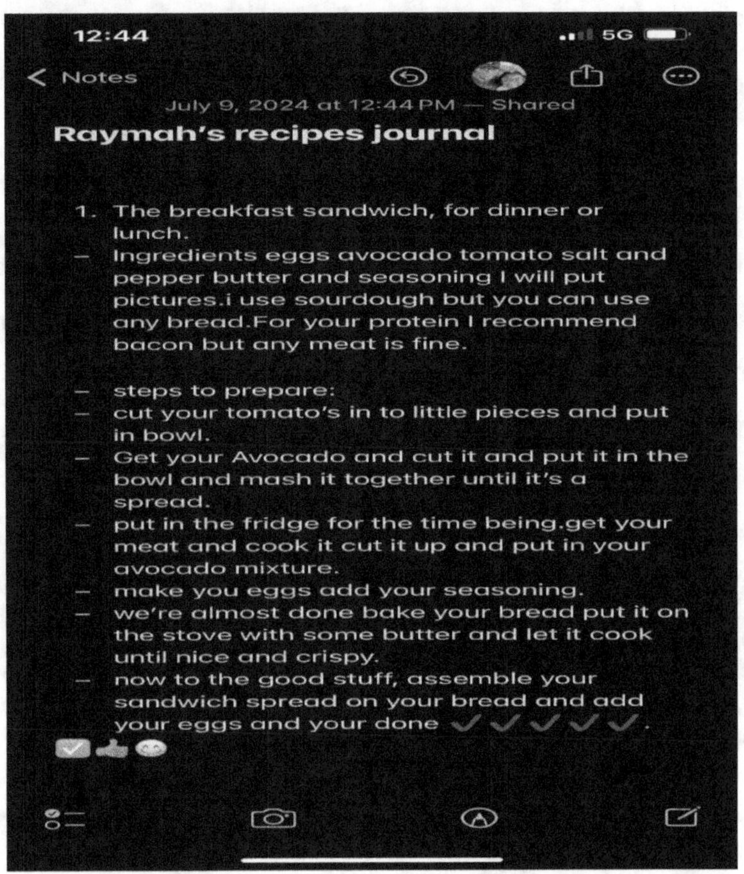

Conclusion

Living a healthy life with diabetes is all about making mindful choices. Through my experiences and research, I've learned that eating well doesn't have to be boring or restrictive. I hope these recipes and activities inspire you to explore new flavors and maintain a balanced lifestyle. Remember, it's not just about the food we eat but the habits we build and the joy we find in our daily activities.

Stay healthy and happy cooking!

Acknowledgments

A big thank you to my family for supporting me in every way possible, especially my mom for being my biggest cheerleader and my stepmother for teaching me about dietary restrictions. To my dad for our yoga sessions and my stepdad for our fishing trips, you all make my life rich and full.

About the Author

Raymah Bryant is a dynamic 11-year-old who excels in school and life. She is passionate about healthy living, loves playing volleyball and dancing, and enjoys creating delicious and nutritious meals. Raymah is an advocate for mindfulness and a role model for other young people managing diabetes. She believes in the power of good habits and strives to inspire others through her journey.

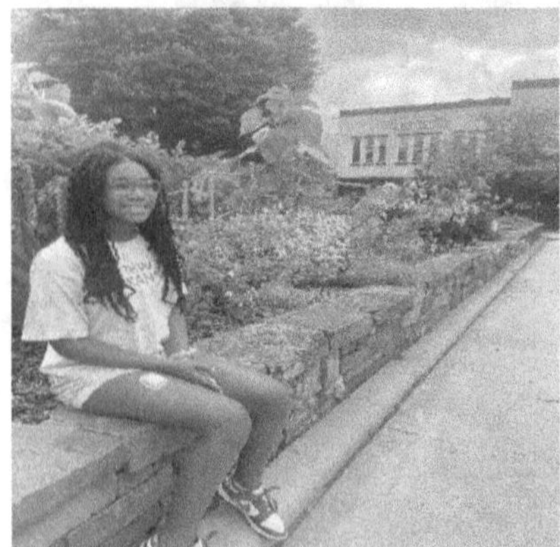

www.ingramcontent.com/pod-product-compliance
Lightning Source LLC
Chambersburg PA
CBHW050800250726
48662CB00005B/2327